ACKNOWLEDGMEN

MW00335036

Grateful acknowledgment is made to the following journals in which these poems appear (sometimes in earlier forms):

American Letters & Commentary: "Fortune Teller Redux" and
    "Gone"
Blackbird: "Coffey Still"
The Briar Cliff Review: "The World's Longest-Running
    Scientific Experiment, 2010" and "Inclined Plane"
burntdistrict: [   ] ("So When Tomorrow Folds")
Midway Journal: "And No Machine Can Have New Ideas"
New Orleans Review: "How Simple Machines Work," "Klein
    Bottle," "Leyden Jar," and "Ratchet"
North Dakota Quarterly: "Franklin Bells"
The NonBinary Review: "Cento: *Frankenstein*, by Mary Shelley"
One Sentence Poems: "Faraday Cage"
Painted Bride Quarterly: "The Frankfurt Kitchen"
Rogue Agent: "Wankel Engine"
Salt Hill: "Moving Bodies Through Direct Contact"
South Dakota Review: "Wedgwood Porcelain"
Sugar House Review: "Wheel & Axle" and "Cento: 'Instinct,'
    by Lester Del Rey"
Tinderbox Poetry Review: "Strand Beast"
Western Humanities Review: "Archimedes Screw," "Diesel Engine,"
    and "Ferris Wheel to the Fun House"

"How Simple Machines Work," "Wheel & Axle," and "Diesel
Engine" were also published in the chapbook *The Verge of Thirst*
(South Dakota State Poetry Society, 2013).

THANKS

I'd like to thank everyone who read these poems, and the manuscript as a whole, in the early stages. That list includes, but is not limited to, Jacqueline Osherow, Katharine Coles, Kathryn Stockton, Barry Weller, Randy Stewart, Julie Gonnering Lein, Esther Lee, Anne Jamison, Danielle Endres, Greg Forter, Max Mueller, Bob Goldberg, Rachel Marston, Valerie Wetlaufer, Brenda Sieczkowski, Shira Dentz, and Robert Glick. I am especially appreciative to the members of the Dakota Women's Poetry Workshop for their help: Darla Biel, Heidi Czerwiec, Jeanne Emmons, Lindy Obach, Pen Pearson, Marcella Remund, Christine Stewart, and Norma Wilson. Thank you to David Ray Vance for suggesting the formatting and title for "Fortune Teller Redux," though I have recreated and modified the design here; any inconsistencies are my own. Thanks to Anne Kelly, Natanya Pulley, Jeylan Yassin, Shelly Tarpley, the Huebner Gloege family, Vince Redder, Erin Desmond, and Clint Desmond for particular kindnesses lately. Special thanks to Andrew Breitenbach, Theodore Breitenbach, James Duffey, Virginia Duffey, and Susan Steward. For their kind words, thanks to Lee Ann Roripaugh and James Allen Hall. For selecting my manuscript, thanks to everyone at The Word Works. Thank you for this prize. I am truly fortunate to have been welcomed into such a supportive group of writers. More thanks than I can express to my editor, Nancy White.

Thank you to Dakota Wesleyan University.

I'd like to thank the Tanner Humanities Center and the National Endowment for the Arts for financial support that allowed me to write and revise these poems.

SIMPLE MACHINES

Also by Barbara Duffey:

I Might Be Mistaken

SIMPLE MACHINES

Barbara Duffey

WINNER OF THE 2015 WASHINGTON PRIZE

THE WORD WORKS
WASHINGTON D.C.

THE WORD WORKS
P.O. Box 42164
Washington, D.C. 20015
editor@wordworksbooks.org

Cover art: "Talking Hand 7," silkscreen. Annika McIntosh.
Cover design: Susan Pearce Design
Author photograph: Virginia Duffey

LCCN: 2016933936
ISBN: 978-0-915380-99-2

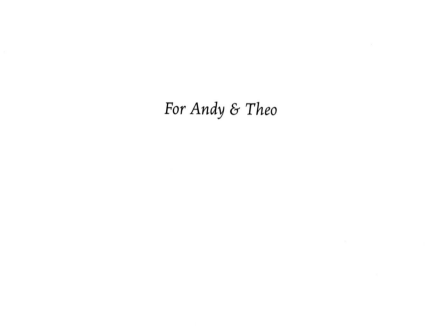

For Andy & Theo

CONTENTS

Any device that transfers a force from the point where it is applied to another point where it is used, is a machine (from a Latin word meaning "invention" or "device"). The lever does this, since a force applied on one side of the fulcrum can lift a weight on the other side; it does this in so uncomplicated a fashion that it cannot be further simplified. It is therefore an example of a simple machine.

...Virtually all the more complicated machines devised and used by mankind until recent times have been merely ingenious combinations of two or more of these simple machines. These machines depend upon the motions and forces produced by moving bodies through direct contact.

—*Understanding Physics*, Isaac Asimov

Our machines are disturbingly lively; we ourselves, frighteningly inert.

—"The Cyborg Manifesto," Donna Haraway

A poem is a small (or large) machine made of words.

—"The Wedge," William Carlos Williams

WHEEL & AXLE

We did nothing on a whim. The friction
of the multiplying moment pulled my
guide, my wagon, to a stream of thimble-
tears until he took my hand and kissed me
when bidden. Love had winched us in from the
wet swarf ground out by the rack-and-pinion
planet, so here we were in front of the
nave and the assembly. We had been clods
in the differential, and now we were
driving an axis of belly and nose.
Aren't we all just hubs housing helical
slave drivers? We wanted our gyroscope
spinning out like a spur-wheel on track,
our little linch-pin, as soon as possible.

DIAGNOSIS: DIMINISHED OVARIAN RESERVE

A bio-alarm activates:
my small stock of old eggs pools
in my body-root,

cools eggs' heels in the pits
of follicles who would have
nurtured my eggs, pulled them

out of my ovaries, into
my game womb. Alas, I am
a poor responder, even

to Follicle Stimulating Hormone.
My blood is like milk
gone off too soon,

retired early on investments
gone bad against the signs. Yet
I reincrease my bet.

[   ]

So when tomorrow folds
in on itself like an ache
I'll visit your voice in the
nest of my want, your shelter.
Baby—please need me shorn
and scalded, needled. I shut myself
down to let science take over your
outset, my makeshift tiny specimen.

Reader, I write to you as a cyborg,
someone with the electronic *Oxford
English Dictionary* attached at her
knuckles. I asked about my machine-mom.
I researched machines in books, finding those
with names that indicated they could be
ancestors. Eponyms. I conducted
an Advanced Search in the *OED* with
the machine-names; the resulting words, which
all contained the machine-names in their
definitions, I listed, avoiding
using any other words, until they
ordered themselves into family missives.

HOW SIMPLE MACHINES WORK

1. *You will never get more energy out of a system than you put into it.*
2. *You will never get as much energy out of a system as you put into it.*

—Utah State University
Junior Engineering Workshop

Rain on a neighbor's shutters, the sound of
learning someone else is pregnant. About

the air, it hung loose as a pinafore,
a thumbed pocket with a grain inside. When

the moon was white as my pall and dog-chained
to dry land, it seemed easier to pitch

my tent alone than bind my body to
you, spoiler pitman, and your paper ribs,

your steam-engine muscle, your Rube Goldberg
romance. But when I maroon my mule self

you always winch me back, even though you
lose heat to friction every time the rope
rubs against the spool as it's wound and wound.

MOVING BODIES THROUGH DIRECT CONTACT

It happened in that soft time lived
between blinks, the small look-my-way, the null
when you were gone. Your return, a scant
rescue, the matter of your touch

Void on an ash-wisp of a
day, I, lead-like, re-clasped my back. Stuttered
something, something tangent. To get some
distance from the pressure of your mouth

You pitched penetrance as an idea,
a remote projection of your skin
on my skin in the space between us—you
radiated into the night's field

An us, a double blood: *Any*
device that transfers a force from the point
where it is applied to another
point where it is used, is a machine.

THE FRANKFURT KITCHEN

First, man had a
kitchen. For a
long time, it was
the only room.
It was bachelor
balm, it was stick-
stick-stock, it was
a family
sugar summer,
all nigh as God
when there are
just four walls. Then
after the war,
in its smoke-jack
world, there became
other, younger
rooms, and no room
for them there in
Germany. So
a lady made
a kitchen halved
like an oyster,
a kitchen cell,
a cook-alley.
There were many
and they purred right,
scarcely as wide
as a skillet.
Let us rejoice

in the spoon-space,
in the platter
cabinet, in the
penny-ouncer
tin-plate rice bin,
from the root, the
room, the roof, we
mouth our prayers in
their ample air,
standing by the
window in the
saucepan sun.

WEDGWOOD PORCELAIN

—With a line adapted from geoscientist Dannie Hidayat

Basalt black as engine bodies, honey,
outside in the marble moonlight, and we're
settling in like a mortar to a match—
slipping open all the seals to raise our
kitchen out of boxes, the tile cold
as old tobacco in a barn, a vase,
a bamboo cane, a pestle made of bone.
If you live with a volcano, it's wise
to watch it closely—the soil is fertile,
but it breathes hot hurricanes of ash. You
enamel me, my sulfur, my biscuit.

MASON JAR

Fetch me an air baby,
the kind who can live without

soil, like certain ferns. The
peculiar kind whose roots

sent puddling will find me
mellow as

a mountain, as an olive
pressed to oil. I am

a trap sealed with a
screw, charge self-set to off.

*

They say the ice-bird
got its name from its call,

the sound of stones sent skidding
across a frozen pond.

*

Embryos can induct
electricity in

growing cells. If a baby
could pick, why not me?

I'm like ice; my calling
is preserving.

KLEIN BOTTLE

*—A single-sided bottle with no boundary whose inside
is its outside*

The baby, the lady, the naked
plate, an open hand, a greenback,

mint muddled in juleps. To pass
the porter, to go out, is to go in,

one-sided plague of presence, his
Möbius in four-dimensioned glass

teases you, it's so impossible
to imagine that baby was inside her.

ARCHIMEDES SCREW

—A pump made of a screw in a pipe

A cochlea turned in cylindrical casing,
lifting river snowmelt to the mill-pool, wraps

the waterline round its single finger
until the polder's dry enough for planting.

Take stock of how we pitch fertility
into the swamp with brutish efficiency.

We are the people of spiral and lever—
we press *impossible* to powder.

THE WORLD'S LONGEST-RUNNING SCIENTIFIC EXPERIMENT, 2010

—A clock driven by temperature variations

Despite not being wound since 1864,
      the Beverly Clock tells time with a diaphragm
            it keeps in an air-tight box; temperature changes

move the mechanism enough to jar each tick-
      tock into motion, turning warm winds into prayer
            posts and play hours, tea dates and bed offices.

When the narrow morning lifts, a lonely motion
      yokes me to these dips and draws so a prodigal's
            constancy can measure out midwinter midnights—

I'll look for you in the wild yellow fields of
      spring and the heat we'll give off will vibrate vesper air;
            let the wren complain if he missed his song hour.

WANKEL ENGINE

—A rotary engine

You say all engines move suspiciously alike,
each piston in its shaft. Must we
build our world in metaphors
of ourselves? I ask if you've heard

of the rotary engine—a triangle twirling
in an oval, opening and closing
its valves, intake, compression, ignition,
exhaust—each triangle-turn condenses the mix
of air and gas in each dwindling chamber
until the spark plug lights it,
spins the triangle back around.

Nothing in nature works like this.
It is banned from some races:
It takes longer to redline,
has none of the most at-risk parts,
no crankshaft or connecting rods.

In that way, you say, it sounds like you.
You wink closed the valve of your eye
as what's behind ignites.

FRANKLIN BELLS

—Bells that chime from the build-up and release of static electricity

A fire-struck sky
and a wind of wires

zap metal hollows
as the clapper hits

one then the other,
charge, release, recharge,

rattle and recoil.
But you and I are

the mellow octave
between *walk* and *stop*.

To tremble is to
strike in double-time—

we're mercury-melt,
paint-dry, grass-grow slow.

LEYDEN JAR

*—A device that stores static electricity between two
electrodes on the inside and outside of a jar*

A charge in glass armature excites like
a drug, like mica glints, like the pith of
a tingle in decay, but when discharged,
the jar meets the world's impedance as a
test-kitchenful of home economists
measuring water in arcane units.
Take yourself to an island and forget
there was ever someone who'd reject you—
close plates mean high voltage, charges equal
but opposite, held apart: a spark
never meant to arc between them.

DIESEL ENGINE

Your airless chutter, your cold consumption,
your push-and-pull, your push-button super-
charge, turbocharger, is not native to
my nose, my mothballed crawler, my purchase
on the underslung world. Mine is inertia,
oil burners, the ring road, gray priming,
scavenging rigid heat. You outdrive me.

LEVER & WEDGE

Interrogate your foot on the crow-bar,
this Lewis & Clark-ing of the unlocked
underneath. We had straight-shot steady-heads
until you looked for hand- and foot-slots in
what used to rest in peace, be decided.
You keep exerting your undue forces;
I'd like to think our own ground is tolling,
un-mechanic, in gears of its own, shorn.

MONKEY WRENCH

Metal molded to the shape of need:
a tight nut released from its bolt.

FERRIS WHEEL TO THE FUN HOUSE

O, my frenemy under the big oyster moon
in your pageant of red-light queens with their rubber

skin, play your medicine for landing patrons whose
wings at camber angles tail lovers, evening

landings. I am lamentably demountable,
living in the midway at any of fifty

state fairs, any early summer nonce carnival
that hangs the smell of roasted nut meat in the air.

Teach me how to keep them strapped in their gondolas
longer than two minutes, as you trap them in your

false turns and warped mirrors, your shifting floors and clown-
laughs to organ fugues. Teach me how to look away

from the water's hypnosis, my spinning likeness,
to ask the dismantlers to give me quarter,
a rudder in the earthquaking, splashed-up future.

FARADAY CAGE

—An enclosure of conducting material

You, my keeper, my mooring
against a blast of blue—

You block
the electro-magnetic

fields, return me
ultimate white

weighing
a capacity

with air

RATCHET

A dog impulse is an old thing to pass
through—a bit, a catch, a clack, a pawl that
stops the cog from turning back. Like time, a
ratchet reaches forward, only; your hand
in its easy offering, I left once
to rattle the air empty as a plate—
that pinion-latch must mean I mean it still.

COFFEY STILL

—A two-column alcohol still

I relish the peavine summer with its
new mouse muzzles and rabbits in the grass,
its whiskey in the mist of a warming
morning rank with the thick world, pink roses
pricked red, and the rest that will outlast us.

"No scientist has ever been able to make a machine as neat and light as your body that could do even half the things your body does. And no machine can have new ideas, or make jokes, or change its mind—or have babies."

—Judy Hindley, *How Your Body Works: A Trip Inside the Body Machine*, 1975.

I read Hindley's book as a child.

[   ]

splitting cells
for a kid machine,
my Icarus belly
ghost-empty

AND NO MACHINE CAN HAVE NEW IDEAS

*—An erasure of Dubois, D.M. (2008). "New trends in
computing anticipatory systems: Emergence of artificial
conscious intelligence with machine learning natural
language."* AIP Conference Proceedings, 1051(1), 25-32.

A memory of past values: We shall
allow M and S to be coupled. We
shall restrict ourselves—we cannot control
any errors. It could provoke. This is
a drastic condition. Purely, fully

anticipatory respiration
and heartbeat, natural evolution
of the life and species. An awareness
of wanting the act. Veto it. At that
moment, there is no place for knowing. The
final time, something new must be added.

My answer was collapse. I, like a bird,
do not know if the cat is dead. Issue:

the dice and the coin have no memory.

CENTO: "INSTINCT," BY LESTER DEL REY

The old brain in his chest even seemed
to think better now. It was good to have
a new body. A good body. How good
it was to be alive and to be a
robot. But the old worries: They were no
nearer re-creating Man than they had
been when they started. They began dissecting
the body of the female failure,
the reason behind the lack of success.
How well do you know your history?
I mean about the beginning.

OR MAKE JOKES

—*An erasure of Suslov, I.M. (2007). "Computer model
of 'a sense of humour'. I. General algorithm."* Cornell
University arXiv Database. <arxiv.org/abs/0711.2058>

A false quickening
pleasure, bare, early
stages of the present.

Lie still. Exaggerated
movements, parodies
of the deviation, invariably

rejected (*that is why the
tickling should be done by
another person*). We begin

the formulation. Suppose
a dictionary family?
In correspondence to images

stored in memory.
Chosen. Meaningful.
Has a form of a tree,

transmitted to the
consciousness of the man.
The probabilistic

makes mistakes inevitable.
Desirable. The man
perceives the low signal:

Dangerous. Probable.
Or he is not tempted.
Nervous laughter.

INSEMINATION

I, pre-progeny. My
livability.

A
gamete, then
a head,
again.

Again, I
support
test-tube you.

Last
       straw
last
       prize,

the best infectant,

a head
again

OR CHANGE ITS MIND

—An erasure of Vernor Vinge's article "The Coming Technological Singularity: How to Survive in the Post-Human Era" (1993)

Wake up, intimate. Let me
make inventions, "what if's" in our heads.

We are the lower
animals. Our models must
be discarded as we move
beyond control, runaway
humankind, the tools of
rabbits—

lots of false starts in
creative endeavors. Our
artifacts suddenly rise.
My rampant optimism
avoided competence, but
nothing would ever "wake up,"
embed "helpful advice," run
a dog mind unfettered. So
hard to articulate, some
kindness, the right guiding
nudge.

     Mutualism
is the great driving force in
evolution. Note that I,
wild organism, break
the fine-scale architecture
of vision.

We need vastly
more animal success—a

little scary on its face,
based on fang and talon.

And
suppose we could gain our most
extravagant hopes, new life

growing—pieces of ego
can be copied and merged,
the size of nature
brought to be.

CENTO: *FRANKENSTEIN,* BY MARY SHELLEY

It was with these feelings that I began
the creation of a human being.
Physical secrets. Have you drunk also
of the intoxicating draught? I had
desired it with an ardour that far
exceeded moderation, to forget
myself and my ephemeral, because
human, sorrows. The wounded deer was but
a type of me. Whence, I often ask my-
self, did the principle of life proceed?
An inanimate body. For this I
had deprived myself of rest and health. My
work drew near a close; now every day showed
how well I had succeeded. I became
myself capable of bestowing

—OR HAVE BABIES

—*An erasure of Zykov, V., Mytilianaios, E., Adams, B., and Lipson, H. (2005). "Self-reproducing machines: A set of modular robot cubes accomplish a feat fundamental to biological systems." Nature, 435 (7039), 163-164.*

Here we create detached,
functional copies of breaks
and joins. Faces change
their faces, governed by
time and contact events.

A supply of material lifting.
How hurdle a continuum
well-defined for others?

Exceedingly high.
For animals, mechanical.
This could be useful.

STRAND BEAST

—After Theo Jansen

The wolves bind my belly-cast, my body
a fox-draw, primitive milkground.

The green-eyed ocean had its run
of my skeleton, trumpeted

up any salient sorrow,
until the dog-girl lunged out spring.

Then I was three strangers. I was
wire in the skin, I was put

out of number. I moved a little
like water. I came back to my

seat on the stoop: everything covered
the devil and rocked sorrow out.

—OR HAVE BABIES

—*An erasure of Wallich, P. (2009). "Hands on: A self-made machine." IEEE Spectrum, 46 (1), 24-25.*

I don't etch;
I build. I would very
much like to need humans,

to work a cup, a coat
hook, a door handle, as
well as making print.

THE BODY MACHINE

*—An erasure of Falk, T.H., Guirgis, M., Power, S., Blain, S.,
and Chau, T. (2010). "On the use of peripheral autonomic
signals for binary control of body-machine interfaces."*
Physiological Measurement, 31, 1411-1422.

Signals work
skin, silent
startle. Access to
eye, tongue
gesture and speech.
Muscle.

          A non-functional
          body.

                    To translate
                    intent into actions,
                    body-machine
                    interfaces.

             Dog,
             glass,
             door imagery.

Interbeat
intervals,
contraction
of the chest.

             Deviated from likelihood.

                     True
                     negatives.

—OR HAVE BABIES

—*An erasure of Groß, R., et al. (2009). "Towards an
autonomous evolution of non-biological physical organisms."*
Lecture Notes in Computer Science (including
subseries Lecture Notes in Artificial Intelligence and
Lecture Notes in Bioinformatics), *173-180.*

Dedicated to stimuli,

The world is populated
by physical objects

a connection, part of a same. Respond
day or night, hard-wired to *replicate*

The day regions were separated
by equally-sized night regions

to assemble from scratch
a human, the body automatic.

THE WORLD'S LONGEST-RUNNING SCIENTIFIC EXPERIMENT, 2014

—Parnell's pitch-drop experiment

The pitch-drop hanging full,
fat, in accord with air,
the funnel mouthed the black

pearl down, one finally
fell in the beaker with
the eight previous drops,

and stuck; the professor
removed the beaker, the
brittle bitumen snapped

and the ninth drop was done,
spun from the funnel's throat
in arabesque through the

states of matter, fourteen
years in slowest free-fall.
We, the rabblement of

kind words and bad pairings,
somehow did not have to
wait so long in our stint

with the butt shots and blood
draws, the distillation,
subcutaneous, of

hormone cocktails, parceled
optimism meted
month by month. Parnell died

before the third drop fell,
his successor died ere
the ninth; a parable

for perseverance or
a warning that our dreams,
met or not, outlive us.

INCLINED PLANE

I'm a non-scientist—
I shoot this obliquely:

If you screw and screw with
still no body housed in

your overfolded frame,
you will be subject to

platitudinism:
it's not in God's plan, it

wasn't meant to be, you
wouldn't be given more

than you could jinny down
that radical needle

of motion, kinetic
thrust of time, perhaps your

house twists with truncated
genes. Yet I felt my child

like a compass needle
in night navigation

slanting, right as polar
pull, some slip-way in my

tilt, his runabout nerves.
I semi-shelved him till

the doctor and his art,
that acceleration

of my milk and family,
somehow returned me to

subsistent skin. In a
word, he was weight, he was

strong, pitched, wedged in there, mine
and striking with small soles.

I want you to be a cyborg too, Reader,
and have made you some Poem Machines
you can use to create a cog unity
for composition. You might need scissors,
and, if you have one, a bone folder.

The professor then desired me "to observe; for he was
going to set his engine at work." The pupils, at his
command, took each of them hold of an iron handle,
whereof there were forty fixed round the edges of the
frame; and giving them a sudden turn, the whole
disposition of the words was entirely changed. He then
commanded six-and-thirty of the lads, to read the
several lines softly, as they appeared upon the frame;
and where they found three or four words together
that might make part of a sentence, they dictated to
the four remaining boys, who were scribes. This work
was repeated three or four times, and at every turn, the
engine was so contrived, that the words shifted into
new places, as the square bits of wood moved upside
down.

—Jonathan Swift, *Gulliver's Travels*

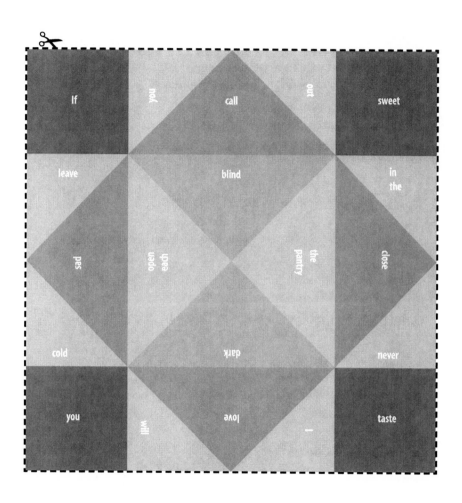

FOLDING INSTRUCTIONS

1. Go find a machine
   that will enlarge the image
   200%. Cut out the square.

2. Hold sheet with image
   facing you.

3. Put "if" in your left hand
   and "taste" in your right;
   fold in half
   so those corners touch,
   then unfold.

4. Fold across opposite diagonal
   so that "you" and "sweet" touch,
   then unfold.

5. Place on table blank side up
   and fold all corners to center.

6. Flip over.
   You should see
   "call/blind," "love/dark," etc.

7. Fold all four corners to center,
   so you see "you out," "in the cold," etc.

8. Flip over,
   so you see the four flaps:
   "If," "you," "taste,"
   and "sweet."

9. Put right index and middle fingers
        under two adjacent flaps
            while simultaneously
                    inserting
                left index and middle fingers
            into the other two flaps.
        Fold the object in on itself,
    forming a shape like a flower bud.

FORTUNE TELLER REDUX

If you taste sweet
leave in the cold never
sad
open each

Sweet if you taste
I will you out
call blind

sweet in the close never taste
out the pantry I
call blind dark love
you open each will
if leave sad cold you

taste sweet if you
leave in the never cold
close the pantry

GONE

swept   against   my jaw

                        your shoulder
        felt like

    falling   your body   your arm

     on the crown of my head
                       which   burned

    we were   both supposed to   keep it up

   you were a weight   we were supposed to see

                       joy

the Phoenix

GONE

you swept   against   my jaw

    first night

     watched   your shoulder

       you felt like the

    happy   falling   your body and your arm

     on the crown of my head

            which burned

         as if it

   were   a boat we were both supposed to   keep it up

the whole two   you were a weight I was   we were supposed to

    see everything   bigger than   joy

we separated   the Phoenix   lovers

    the one

GONE

you swept your thumb against   my jaw   your   cup

that first night in my kitchen

     I watched   behind your shoulder

           you felt like the inside

I was so happy I kept falling

                 I could sit your body and your arm

         on the crown of my head   my pageboy

in the wind   which burned

          hunger   as if it

were next on a boat we were both supposed to paddle,
                           keep it up
the whole two miles. you were a weight I was proud of.

         we were supposed to see dolphins,

but   everything was bigger than   joy. when

we separated   the Phoenix   could think of   lovers   the one

the one

STRETCH POEM:
SO WHEN TOMORROW FOLDS

So frightening when tomorrow the doctor folds

my body in on itself I'll wish like an ache for
you. I'll visit your crib, hear your voice in the made-up,

nest of my belly, my want, your Icarus shelter.
Baby— ghost, please need me empty shorn

bald and scalded, needled. That's how I shut myself out
quiet down to let science whisper you, take over your glass

outset, splitting cells my makeshift kid machine, you tiny specimen,

FOLDING INSTRUCTIONS

This time you will need to see as well as hear the steps. Go to **http://www.wordworksbooks.org/origami-instructions** to watch the video that will make all clear.

SO WHEN TOMORROW FOLDS

So frightening when tomorrow the doctor folds
my body in on itself. I'll wish like an ache
for you. I'll visit your crib, hear your voice in the made-up
nest of my belly, my want, your Icarus shelter.
Baby-ghost, please need me empty, shorn
bald and scalded, needled. That's how I shut myself out,
quiet down to let science whisper you, take over your glass
outset, splitting cells, my makeshift kid-machine, you tiny
                                        specimen.

DEFENSE MECHANISM

Running a sector of myself
free of the mind-brain interface,
like setting up a pantomime screen:

it seems a defense, a negative,
but is a charge, a projection
of a life's motions, the undoing
of the *nom de théâtre* I gave

to each issue. I credit
the iron-rich earth where I played
as a child, the nickelwork
coincident with my youth—
a cover peremptory, empty
as two hands cupped to form a dog's head.

INTRAUTERINE INSEMINATION BYPASSES THE CERVIX

That small stem—
if you look up
"intrauterine"
in the *OED*,
you'll see it's mentioned in
definitions of words such
as "non-" and "missed" and "blood-staunching."
What made me maternal was
in a catheter laced
through my cervix, sperm
waiting for my one
good—best!—egg.
Non-missed.

ETERNALLY OPENING ORIGAMI: RELIEF

—*After Paul Jackson's figure "Eternally Opening Origami,"
of which he says, "It is nothing more than the classic
Bird Base, familiar to all experienced folders. What
makes it remarkable is that no one until Takuji
Sugimura of Japan [author of* Living Origami, *1995]
realized that it could perform the addictive dance
described here."*

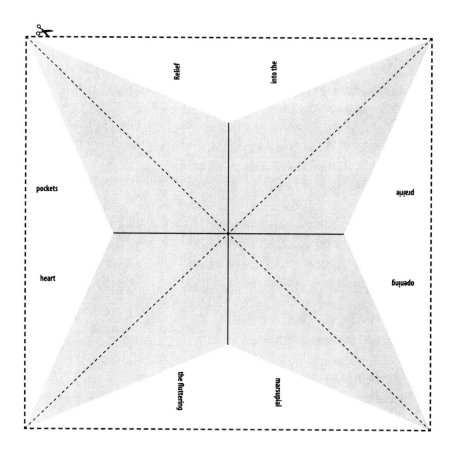

FOLDING INSTRUCTIONS

1. Enlarge and cut
   out the figure
   as before.

2. Fold along the diagonal dotted
   lines so that the blank
   side is visible when you make your fold.
   Unfold.

3. Fold along the solid,
   perpendicular lines so that the printed
   side is visible when you fold.
   Fold all the way across the page
   even though the line does not extend
   all the way. Unfold.

4. Fold the top edge, containing "Relief"
   and "into the," down to meet
   the bottom edge. The printed side
   should now be showing.

5. Hold the bottom-left and
   bottom-right corners.

6. Bring the corners together; the paper
   should form a tilted square
   with its hinged tip
   pointing up.

7. Flatten the figure into a square.

8. Hold the figure so the closed
   corner is at the top and
   the open corner is at the bottom.
   Fold both sides (just the top layer)
   in along the gray lines to meet the middle line,
   making a kite shape.
   It should read
   "prairie / into the / heart / the fluttering."

9. Fold down the top gray triangle
   over the kite wings.

10. Pull the top side
    kite wing triangles
    back out, restoring
    the square shape.

11. Hold just the top layer
    of the bottom corner
    of your square/kite.
    Lift it upwards.

12. Bring it all
    the way up so
    that the kite wing triangles
    fold inward.

13. Flatten those elongated side triangles.
    Now you have a tall diamond.

14. Turn the figure over and repeat
    steps 8-13 on that side.

15. Hold the figure so that
    the open ends
    are on top and the lettering
    is upside-down.

16. Hold each open end
    in one of your hands.
    Move your hands away from each other
    and down, so that the open ends go down
    as the closed ends rise.
    Make sure that you
    pull both out and down at the same time;
    if you pull just out, and not down,
    the paper will lock and make it
    impossible for you
    to move the ends
    down.

17. Continue until your original
    top ends are now
    at the bottom.

18. Transfer your hands
    to the new top
    ends and repeat
    steps 16 and 17.
    Read the poem on each
    side each time
    you repeat. As you open it again and again,
    the paper will soften and open more easily each time.

RELIEF

Relief opening
into the prairie

Marsupial pockets
the fluttering heart

Marsupial opening
the fluttering prairie

Relief pockets
into the heart

THE FUN HOUSE REPLIES
TO THE FERRIS WHEEL

Like the arabesques of apples falling
into their barrel, the percussion of
their heavy globes blonk-blonking on wood. Like
a baby alludes to an animal,
its meaty laugh, its piss, its ribs, its skin.
Like the street, sticky with stuff.

Like a wound action swinging the clock's arm,
I generate the ghosts of dreams, the jests
merry in your highest heart, body bank
of our machine mothers, fair engines of
faces milking mischief for all it's worth.
You pivot, I puzzle; the rain wakes the ticketholders.

I, ETERNALLY OPENING

O, small   pen,
                stop to my

waste,

the decline of all
my ideas.
You,

baby,   little   poke,
world,   begin me

        my case
a corner of a lip
        tipped up,
this time.

ABOUT THE AUTHOR

Barbara Duffey is a 2015 NEA Literature Fellow in poetry and the author of the full-length poetry collection *I Might Be Mistaken* (Word Poetry, 2015), as well as the chapbooks *The Circus of Forgetting* (dancing girl press, 2013) and *The Verge of Thirst* (South Dakota State Poetry Society, 2013). Her poems have appeared in such publications as *Blackbird*, *Prairie Schooner*, *Western Humanities Review*, and *Best New Poets 2009*, and her prose in *CutBank* and *The Collagist*. She holds a PhD from the University of Utah, an MFA from the University of Houston, and a BA *summa cum laude* from the University of Southern California. She is an assistant professor of English at Dakota Wesleyan University and lives in Mitchell, S.D., with her husband and son. You can find her online at barbaraduffey.com and on Twitter @BarbaraNDuffey.

ABOUT THE ARTIST

Annika McIntosh is an artist and landscape designer who lives in Seattle. She holds a MS in Landscape Architecture.

ABOUT THE WORD WORKS

The Word Works, a nonprofit literary organization, publishes contemporary poetry and presents public programs.
Other imprints besides the Washington Prize include the Hilary Tham Capital Collection, the Tenth Gate Prize, and International Editions. A reading period is also held in May.

Monthly, The Word Works offers free literary programs in the Chevy Chase, MD, Café Muse series, and each summer, it holds free poetry programs in Washington, D.C.'s Rock Creek Park. Annually in June, two high school students debut in the Joaquin Miller Poetry Series as winners of the Jacklyn Potter Young Poets Competition. Since 1974, Word Works programs have included: "In the Shadow of the Capitol," a symposium and archival project on the African American intellectual community in segregated Washington, D.C.; the Gunston Arts Center Poetry Series; the Poet Editor panel discussions at The Writer's Center; and Master Class workshops.

As a 501(c)3 organization, The Word Works has received awards from the National Endowment for the Arts, the National Endowment for the Humanities, the D.C. Commission on the Arts & Humanities, the Witter Bynner Foundation, Poets & Writers, The Writer's Center, Bell Atlantic, the David G. Taft Foundation, and others, including many generous private patrons.

An archive of artistic and administrative materials is housed in the Washington Writing Archive of the George Washington University Gelman Library. The Word Works is a member of the Council of Literary Magazines and Presses and its books are distributed by Small Press Distribution.

wordworksbooks.org

The Washington Prize

Nathalie F. Anderson, *Following Fred Astaire*, 1998

Michael Atkinson, *One Hundred Children Waiting for a Train*, 2001

Molly Bashaw, *The Whole Field Still Moving Inside It*, 2013

Carrie Bennett, *biography of water*, 2004

Peter Blair, *Last Heat*, 1999

John Bradley, *Love-in-Idleness: The Poetry of Roberto Zingarello*, 1995, 2nd edition 2014

Christopher Bursk, *The Way Water Rubs Stone*, 1988

Richard Carr, *Ace*, 2008

Jamison Crabtree, *Rel[AM]ent*, 2014

B. K. Fischer, *St. Rage's Vault*, 2012

Linda Lee Harper, *Toward Desire*, 1995

Ann Rae Jonas, *A Diamond Is Hard But Not Tough*, 1997

Frannie Lindsay, *Mayweed*, 2009

Richard Lyons, *Fleur Carnivore*, 2005

Elaine Magarrell, *Blameless Lives*, 1991, 2nd edition 2016

Fred Marchant, *Tipping Point*, 1993

Ron Mohring, *Survivable World*, 2003

Barbara Moore, *Farewell to the Body*, 1990

Brad Richard, *Motion Studies*, 2010

Jay Rogoff, *The Cutoff*, 1994

Prartho Sereno, *Call from Paris*, 2007, 2nd edition 2013

Enid Shomer, *Stalking the Florida Panther*, 1987

John Surowiecki, *The Hat City After Men Stopped Wearing Hats*, 2006

Miles Waggener, *Phoenix Suites*, 2002

Charlotte Warren, *Gandhi's Lap*, 2000

Mike White, *How to Make a Bird with Two Hands*, 2011

Nancy White, *Sun, Moon, Salt*, 1992, 2nd edition 2010

George Young, *Spinoza's Mouse*, 1996

The Hilary Tham Capital Collection

Mel Belin, *Flesh That Was Chrysalis*
Carrie Bennett, *The Land Is a Painted Thing*
Doris Brody, *Judging the Distance*
Sarah Browning, *Whiskey in the Garden of Eden*
Grace Cavalieri, *Pinecrest Rest Haven*
Cheryl Clarke, *By My Precise Haircut*
Christopher Conlon, *Gilbert and Garbo in Love*
 & *Mary Falls: Requiem for Mrs. Surratt*
Donna Denizé, *Broken like Job*
W. Perry Epes, *Nothing Happened*
Bernadette Geyer, *The Scabbard of Her Throat*
Barbara G. S. Hagerty, *Twinzilla*
James Hopkins, *Eight Pale Women*
Brandon Johnson, *Love's Skin*
Marilyn McCabe, *Perpetual Motion*
Judith McCombs, *The Habit of Fire*
James McEwen, *Snake Country*
Miles David Moore, *The Bears of Paris*
 & *Rollercoaster*
Kathi Morrison-Taylor, *By the Nest*
Tera Vale Ragan, *Reading the Ground*
Michael Shaffner, *The Good Opinion of Squirrels*
Maria Terrone, *The Bodies We Were Loaned*
Hilary Tham, *Bad Names for Women*
 & *Counting*
Barbara Louise Ungar, *Charlotte Brontë, You Ruined My Life*
 & *Immortal Medusa*
Jonathan Vaile, *Blue Cowboy*
Rosemary Winslow, *Green Bodies*
Michele Wolf, *Immersion*
Joe Zealberg, *Covalence*

International Editions

Kajal Ahmad (Alana Marie Levinson-LaBrosse, Mewan
Nahro Said Sofi, and Darya Abdul-Karim Ali Najin,
trans., with Barbara Goldberg), *Handful of Salt*
Keyne Cheshire (trans.), *Murder at Jagged Rock: A Tragedy
by Sophocles*
Yoko Danno & James C. Hopkins, *The Blue Door*
Moshe Dor, Barbara Goldberg, Giora Leshem, eds.,
The Stones Remember: Native Israeli Poets
Moshe Dor (Barbara Goldberg, trans.), *Scorched by the Sun*
Lee Sang (Myong-Hee Kim, trans.), *Crow's Eye View:
The Infamy of Lee Sang, Korean Poet*
Vladimir Levchev (Henry Taylor, trans.), *Black Book of
the Endangered Species*

Other Word Works Books

Karren L. Alenier, *Wandering on the Outside*
Karren L. Alenier, ed., *Whose Woods These Are*
Karren L. Alenier & Miles David Moore, eds.,
Winners: A Retrospective of the Washington Prize
Christopher Bursk, ed., *Cool Fire*
Barbara Goldberg, *Berta Broadfoot and Pepin the Short*
Frannie Lindsay, *If Mercy*
Marilyn McCabe, *Glass Factory*
Ayaz Pirani, *Happy You Are Here*
W.T. Pfefferle, *My Coolest Shirt*
Jacklyn Potter, Dwaine Rieves, Gary Stein, eds.,
Cabin Fever: Poets at Joaquin Miller's Cabin
Robert Sargent, *Aspects of a Southern Story
& A Woman from Memphis*
Nancy White, ed., *Word for Word*

CPSIA information can be obtained
at www.ICGtesting.com
Printed in the USA
LVOW12s1009141016
508775LV00001B/21/P